MAKING YOUR OWN HAND SANITIZER AND DISINFECTANT

DIY Guide With Easy Recipes to Make Your Homemade Hand Sanitizer and Disinfectant

Written By

Noelle Stephens

Contents

Introduction

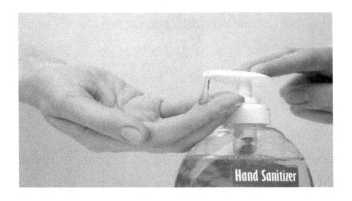

We encounter bacteria and viruses every day, and while many of them are harmless, some of these germs can cause lethal diseases. The introduction of new, and unusual strains of viruses and bacteria today only emphasized the importance of proper hygiene.

Taking extra precautions to protect yourself is crucial, especially if you want to prevent the circulation of contagious diseases.

Unless you have an arsenal of commercial hand sanitizers, finding one today may be almost impossible, especially with the high demand in retail stores. Well, don't fret! There's good news! Although washing your hands is still the most effective way of protecting yourself from germs, you can't always have access to soap and a sink. So how should you protect yourself from here?

According to the Centers for Disease Control and Prevention (CDC), the next best thing is the hand sanitizer.

However, some commercial sanitizers may contain substances that can cause more damage than the germs they protect you from. So if you're looking at an empty bottle of your old hand sanitizer, you don't have to worry. Knowing easy recipes to create your home hand sanitizer from simple ingredients in your kitchen or the local drug store could be essential in protecting you and your loved ones.

Much more, learning how to make your homemade sanitizer saves you money, equips you with the knowledge to protect yourself germs, and, most importantly, gives your sanitizer the smell of your choice.

This isn't a regular hand sanitizer recipe book. Our objective is to provide an extensive overview of different recipes for your homemade hand sanitizer, how to use them, helpful tips on how to stay safe, and so much more.

Let's Dig in!

How exactly do hand Sanitizers work?

Most sanitizer companies boast about how their products kill 99.9% of germs. But how true is this? Is it a myth or a fact? Well, the key component in most hand sanitizers is alcohol. The alcohol in sanitizers kills harmful bacteria and viruses by splitting their proteins or affecting their metabolism. According to

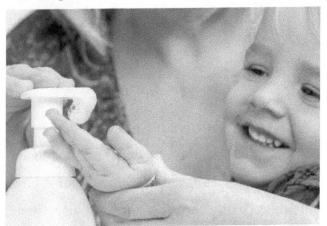

Clinical Microbiology, solutions that contain at least 30% of alcohol can kill some pathogens. The potency of this solution increases with the concentration of alcohol.

For the recipes I am going to teach you, your homemade hand sanitizer should contain more than 60% alcohol to effectively kill most of the germs on your hands.

Hand sanitizers function by removing the external film on your skin.

The effectiveness of your hand sanitizer depends on several factors.

- **Amount of Hand sanitizer**

The amount of hand sanitizer you apply on you determines how effective it will be in fighting off those harmful germs. If you don't use an adequate amount or rub the sanitizer thoroughly — it won't be effective in killing 99.9% of the germs on your hands.

- **Dirty or Grimy Hands**

If your hands are extremely dirty or grimy, your sanitizer won't be as effective as it can be. It works a lot better on clear or mildly dirty hands.

- **Percentage of alcohol composition**

The percentage of alcohol in your sanitizer will determine how effective your sanitizer will be in fighting off germs. If your hand sanitizer contains less than 60% alcohol, it will not be very efficient in removing all the harmful microbes on your hand.

Proper way to use a hand sanitizer

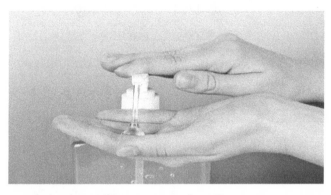

Applying sanitizer your hands seems pretty straightforward — Apply on hands and rub. Still, there's a method for adequate hand sanitizing techniques: Yes, there's a proper way to use a hand sanitizer. You may have been using it wrong. Well, applying your hand sanitizer isn't rocket science. Instead, in less than 30 seconds, you can fight off those germs when you apply it correctly. To make things even easier, I've compiled the process into small and easy steps.

- **Step 1:** First, remove all dirt and greasy stains from your hands.

- **Step 2:** Spray or Apply a dime-size amount on the palm of one hand.

- **Step 3:** Stroke your hands together, ensure you cover all the areas on both hands.

Top tip: Pay close attention to areas between your fingers, and around your fingertips and nails.

- **Step 4:** Rub your hands together for at least 30 seconds to allow your hands to absorb the product completely.

- **Step 5:** Allow your hand sanitizer to dry off completely before you touch any substance.

That's it. Whether you're out in the grocery store, using a public restroom, stuck in traffic, or even using the gas pump, you can sanitize your hand correctly with these 5 easy steps.

How effective is your Homemade Sanitizer?

Before you dive into the recipes, there's one aspect many people ignore – The effectiveness of their homemade hand sanitizer. Since you've made the smart plan to produce your hand sanitizer, there are some factors to consider. Firstly, you must measure your ingredients accurately to ensure your sanitizer maintains its effectiveness. Otherwise, your homemade sanitizer may cause more harm than good. Another essential factor you should consider is the percentage of alcohol. On your old sanitizer bottle, the alcohol may be listed as itemized as ethanol, ethyl alcohol, or isopropyl alcohol. Regardless of the type of alcohol and other ingredients, your sanitizer should have an alcohol percentage of at least 60%. If the concentration falls below 60% [alcohol content], the sanitizer also loses its effectiveness in killing germs.

1.4 Benefits of having a readily available Homemade Sanitizer

Your homemade hand sanitizer can be an invaluable accessory, especially if you're a mother with kids running about and touching almost everything they see. Unfortunately, most sanitizers contain alcohol, and this can be sensitive to their skin.

Well, making your homemade sanitizers with simple, all-natural ingredients that won't irritate and dry out your skin, is within reach.

With just a few essential oils, you can create your own readily available homemade hand sanitizer.

1.5 How to Wash your hands properly

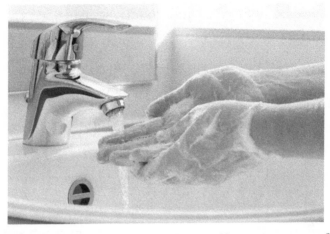

You touch people, your face, office papers, and as you're reading this, maybe you're touching your computer. Regardless of where you touch, germs find their way of accumulating on your hands. Unfortunately, you don't only risk infecting yourself when you touch your eyes, nose, or mouth. You can also spread it to others.

Although it can be far-fetching always to keep your hands free of harmful bacteria and viruses, washing your hands is the best bet to keep your hands germ-free.

Washing your hand correctly, doesn't have to be complicated. I've compiled the technique into 5 easy steps.

Step 1: Switch on your tap and wet your hands (to the wrist). Switch off the tap, and rub an adequate amount of soap.

Top tip: The temperature of the water doesn't matter.

Step 2: Rub your hands together to form a lather. Pay close attention to the backs of your hands, between your fingers, under your nails, and way back up to your wrists.

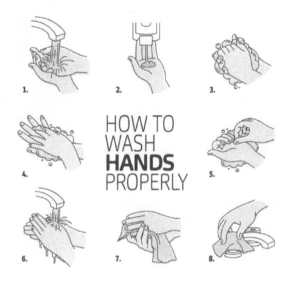

- **Step 3:** Scrub your hands for at least 20 seconds.

Top tip: To make your handwashing process more enjoyable, you can sing a short song to get your timing right.

- **Step 4:** Re-open your tab and rinse your hands thoroughly under clean running water using the same technique.
- **Step 5:** Finally, you can dry your hand using a clean paper towel, a hand dryer, or you can allow your hands to air dry.

Chapter 2

2.1 Homemade Sanitizers

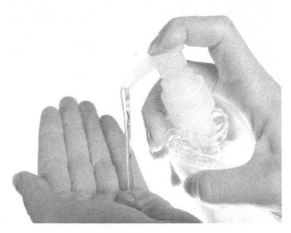

Homemade Sanitizers became even more recognized in 2019 – and appetites for homemade sanitizers don't seem to be slowing down, either. With the high requests for commercial sanitizers, it has become nearly impossible for drug stores and grocery shops to keep up.

Luckily, this isn't necessarily bad news. Besides the suffocating medicinal smell of commercial sanitizers, the dry alcohol in them can also irritate the skin.

Homemade sanitizers are milder for sensitive skin, yet strong enough to use after using public toilets.

Making your homemade sanitizer doesn't have to be expensive or complicated. Instead, to bolster its already impressive advantages, making your sanitizer at home can save you a lot of money and time.

If you're worried about mixing chemicals with chemicals, you probably have the ingredients right in your kitchen cabinet, or worst-case scenario, you may have to visit the local drug store.

The ingredients for your homemade sanitizer are always readily available. As a bonus, with the recipes you're about to learn, you can give your sanitizer the smell of your choice.

2.2 Types of Homemade Sanitizers

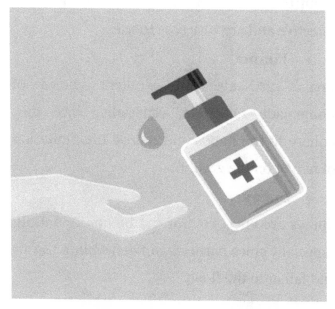

Hand sanitizers come in various forms. However, regardless of what form of homemade sanitizer you choose to make, as long as its alcohol concentration is 60% and above – You have an effective sanitizer.

You can make your sanitizer as either;

- **Gels**

When compared to other types of DIY Sanitizers, Gel sanitizers are more cost-effective and are very easy to use.

- **Foams**

Foams are also an excellent choice of homemade sanitizers, especially since they adhere to the hands and reduce the limitation of falling on the ground.

- **Spray**

Sprays are effective, but can be uneconomical, especially since particles can deflect into the air and fall onto the floor.

2.3 Essential Ingredients for your homemade sanitizer recipes

Just like every great chef has a secret recipe, every homemade sanitizer has its extraordinary ingredient. In this section, you're going to learn about the ingredients you can use for your homemade sanitizer. With these few ingredients, you can unearth and create your custom hand sanitizer. Let's get started!

1) Vinegar

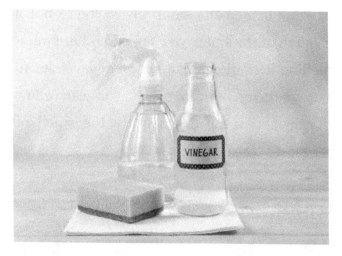

For decades, vinegar has been an invaluable cure for infections, wounds. It also serves as an excellent food preservative and a disinfectant. In recent years, vinegar has proved to be a vital ingredient in sanitizers due to its potent antibacterial property.

It contains antioxidants that repair damaged cells. Vinegar also eliminates harmful bacteria by preventing their multiplication.

The environment-friendly ingredient is usually available in drug stores.

Top tip: I recommend you use white vinegar for your homemade sanitizer. If you're not a huge fan of the smell, you can add other sweet-smelling ingredients like lemon or lavender to your sanitizer. Alternatively, you can allow your hands to air dry because the smell of vinegar disperses easily.

2) Aloe Vera

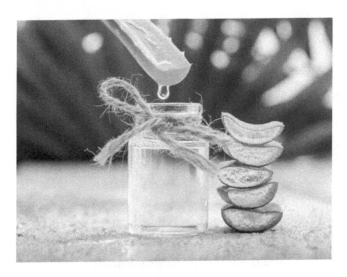

The cell-regenerating Aloe Vera makes a superb addition to our ingredient list and rightly so, this miracle ingredient contains 99% water and about 75 potentially active elements. Aloe's natural healing properties can be credited to its antioxidants, vitamins, enzymes, and antimicrobial properties.

Aloe makes an excellent choice for your homemade sanitizer. Because of its ample water content, Aloe Vera hydrates your hands without leaving the uncomfortable greasy feeling of commercial sanitizers.

3) Alcohol

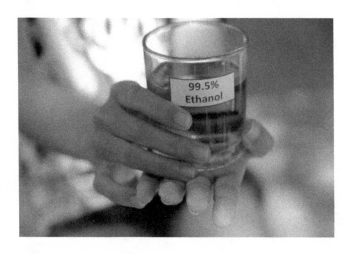

Alcohol is one of the most popular and vital ingredients for your homemade sanitizer. Proof? More than 100 years of practical application. Alcohol works by attacking protein in bacteria, and as a result, kills the cells. However, there's a catch. Using the beer or vodka in your fridge won't be as effective. Your homemade sanitizer needs to have at least 60% alcohol to be effective in fighting germs.

Top tip: I recommend making your sanitizer at least 75% alcohol. If your skin is sensitive and you still find your sanitizer overwhelming, you can add one or two teaspoons of your favorite essential oil to counter this effect.

4) Hydrogen Peroxide

Hydrogen Peroxide makes our ingredient list because of its unbelievable oxidizing power. This robust solution oxidizes when it comes in contact with germs, and causes bacteria to decompose.

Although a Hydrogen peroxide-based sanitizer is very easy to use, it can cause a tingling sensation on contact with the skin.

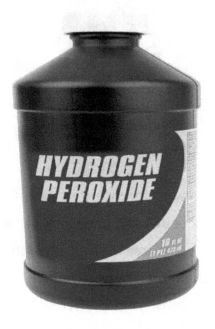

Top tip: If hydrogen peroxide is your preferred ingredient, I recommend you store your hand sanitizer in a dark-colored bottle. Remember to keep it away from sunlight because hydrogen peroxide oxidizes on contact with air.

5) Tea Tree Oil

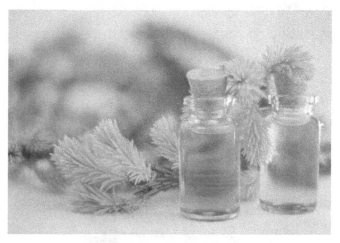

If you're new to the world of essential oils or even a frequent user, then you should know how unique Tea tree oil is, it is a splendid and priceless addition to any collection. Tea tree oil is easily one of our preferred active home ingredients.

Tea tree oil boasts of incredible antiviral, antibacterial, anti-fungal, and anti-inflammatory properties. Since it has potent antiseptic properties, it increases the effectiveness of your homemade hand sanitizer. However, the smell can be pungent.

Top tip: I recommend you properly label your sanitizers because Tea tree oil can be harmful if pregnant women or children ingest it.

Bonus Tip: If your skin is extra sensitive. You can pick one or two essential oils; you don't have to use all of them.

6. Lemon Essential Oil

Lemon essential oil is a natural sweet-smelling antiseptic made from fresh lemons. The essential oil has been around for thousands of years, serving anti-fungal and antibacterial functions.

The lemon essential oil also has brilliant effects on the skin, especially if you're suffering from acne.

Top tip: Although Tea tree oil is a more potent disinfectant, the smell can be stomach-turning. Adding a few drops of Lemon essential oil helps to mask the pungent smell.

7. Winterbloom

The use of winterbloom as a medical disinfectant has been around for decades. Today, due to its practical applications as an antimicrobial agent, it has become an excellent ingredient for making hand sanitizers. In addition to its already impressive qualities, winterbloom also has a small concentration of Alcohol. You should note that the percentage of Alcohol in winterbloom does not meet the 60% requirement to make an effective sanitizer. Nevertheless, winterbloom makes a potent addition when used with other ingredients. I recommend using winterbloom if your skin is sensitive to Alcohol.

Top tip: Depending on your location, winterbloom is also known as witch hazel.

Other vital ingredients you will need for your homemade sanitizer include;

Bowl: To mix your ingredients

Spoon: To stir your ingredients together.

Funnel: To guide your homemade sanitizer into the labeled bottle.

Whisk: Essential Oils don't mix well with water, and usually, stirring may not be enough. You can use the whisk to whip up your recipe into a homogeneous gel.

Plastic bottles: Once you've made the homemade sanitizer of your choice, you will need a safe place to keep it in. I recommend using a transparent bottle with a flip-top. The flip-top makes squeezing out your hand sanitizer almost effortless.

Gloves: You're creating a unique homemade sanitizer to protect yourself from germs, so it's only logical you stay safe when mixing ingredients. Wearing gloves prevents burns and injuries that could result from spills directly on your hand.

Chapter 3

3.1 Recipe 1

Aloe Vera Homemade Hand Gel

Recipe

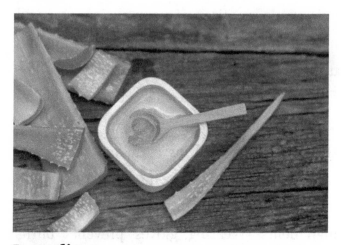

Ingredients

- 1/3 cup of Aloe Vera gel
- 2/3 cup of Alcohol (ethanol or isopropyl alcohol)
- 8-10 drops of cinnamon essential oil
- 8-10 drops of lemon essential oil or lemongrass

- 8-10 drops of tea tree essential oil
- Bowl
- Measuring cup
- Spoon
- Filter
- Clear Bottle
- Labeling materials

Directions

- **1:** Gather all your ingredients on your table
- **2:** Measure your ingredients carefully
- **3**: Mix 2/3 cup of Alcohol with 1/3 cup of Aloe Vera and stir thoroughly.

Top tip: Although it is uncommon knowledge, cracks in your skin can harbor harmful germs. These cracks happen when the ratio of Alcohol and Aloe Vera isn't correctly balanced. Aloe moisturizes your skin and prevents your skin from drying out and cracking, which, in turn, reduces the risk of infection.

Extra substitutions

Cinnamon Essential Oil: The Cinnamon essential Oil is a natural antiseptic that has been used for ions to prevent infection. Adding a few drops of Cinnamon, essential oil will boost your already effective homemade hand sanitizer.

Lemon Essential Oil: Adding a few drops of lemon essential enhances the smell of your homemade sanitizer and masks the unappealing scent of Alcohol.

Glycerol: If you don't have an Aloe plant growing in your backyard, there's an even cheaper alternative – Glycerol. However, your homemade sanitizer may not smell as pleasant.

- **Step 4:** Using your filter, pour your solution into the clear bottle.

3.2 Recipe 2

Tea Tree Oil Recipe

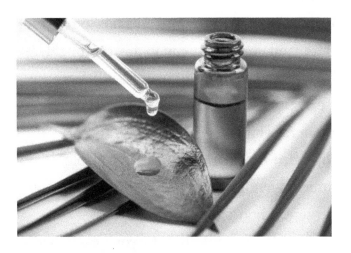

Ingredients to use:

- 10 drops of tea tree oil
- 2/3 cup of Alcohol
- Vitamin E
- 1/3 cup of water
- Bowl
- Measuring cup
- Spoon
- Filter
- Clear Bottle

- Labeling materials

Directions:

Step 1: Pour a 1/3 cup of Alcohol into 150ml water, and use your spoon to mix thoroughly.

Step 2: Add 10 drops of tea tree Oil

Step 3: Add a teaspoon of Vitamin E (Helps soften the skin)

Top tip: Essential Oils are not soluble in water, so naturally, they don't mix well. Ensure you shake thoroughly.

Step 4: Pour carefully into your clear bottle and label correctly.

Bonus Tip: Make sure you keep your Tea tree oil sanitizer in a cool and dark place.

3.3 Recipe 3

Lemon essential oil Recipe

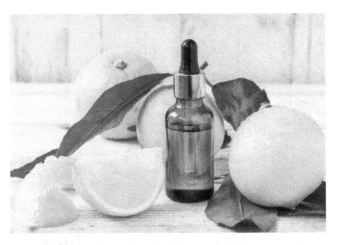

Ingredients to use:

- 8 – 10 drops of lemon essential oil
- 2/3 cup of tap water
- **On request**: 2 -3 drops of cinnamon essential oil
- Bowl
- Measuring cup
- Spoon
- Filter
- Clear Bottle
- Labeling materials

Directions:

Step 1: Pour 1/3 cup of water into your bowl

Step 2: Add 8 – 10 drops of Lemon Essential Oil

Step 3: Mix the solution thoroughly

Top tip: You can add 2-3 drops of Cinnamon essential oil to increase the potency of your homemade sanitizer.

Although cinnamon oil is a powerful antimicrobial agent, it can cause irritation and burns if you use a high concentration. If you notice your skin is irritated, you can tweak the recipe and increase the amount of water.

Bonus point: Water and essential oils don't mix well, so ensure you shake your new hand sanitizer well before you use it.

3.4 Recipe 4

The essential oil of orange Recipe

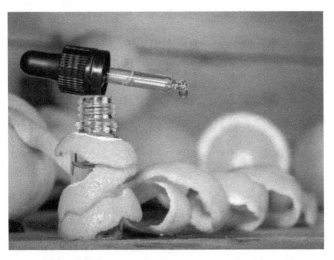

Ingredients to use:

- 5 – 10 drops of essential oil of orange
- 2 drops of Lithium essential oil
- On request: 2 drops of essential oil of thyme
- ½ cup Aloe Vera
- ½ tablespoon of lecithin
- Bowl
- Measuring cup
- Spoon

- Filter
- Clear Bottle
- Labeling materials

Directions

Step 1: Mix your essential oil of orange with 2 drops essential oil of Lithium

On request: Add 2 drops of thyme oil.

Thyme essential oil has established itself as a significant power in fighting antibacterial infections.

Step 2: Add lecithin to the solution and mix the solution thoroughly.

Top tip: Lecithin is usually available at your local drug store.

Step 3: Gradually pour in aloe gel and mix the resulting solution thoroughly.

Top tip: Your hand sanitizer will come out gel-like. Although it can also be used for disinfection, it may not be suitable for use on tables and furniture. I recommend using only on your body.

3.5 Recipe 5

Winterbloom extract Recipe

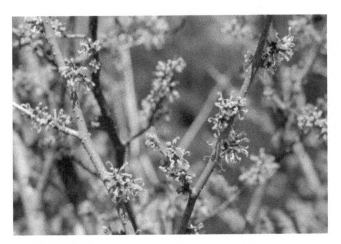

Ingredients:

- 100 ml of winterbloom extract;
- 5 drops of cinnamon essential oil
- 5 drops of essential oils of orange
- 10 drops of Lemon essential oil
- Bowl
- Measuring cup
- Spoon
- Filter
- Clear Bottle
- Labeling materials

On request: To enhance the features of your sanitizer, you can also add 2 tablespoons of Vitamin E (softens skin) or Liquid coconut oil.

Directions

Step 1: Add your winterbloom to a bowl

Step 2: Add 2 tablespoons of vitamin E or coconut oil (Optional)

Step 3: Whisk your solution properly

Step 4: Add Cinnamon and Lemon essential oil and shake again.

3.6 Recipe 6

Lavender Essential Oil Recipe

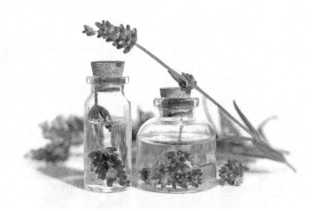

Ingredients:

- 5 drops of Lavender Essential Oil
- 3 tablespoons of Aloe gel
- 5 drops of Cinnamon essential oil
- 10 drops of Tea tree oil
- 5 drops of vitamin E
- 5 drops of Peach seed oil
- Bowl
- Measuring cup
- Spoon
- Filter

- Clear Bottle
- Labeling materials

Directions

Step 1: First, pour Aloe into your bowl, add cinnamon essential oil and tea tree oil.

Step 2: Add 5 drops of Vitamin E, and next, add 5 drops peach seed essential oil.

Step 3: Mix your solution thoroughly.

Step 4: Finally, add your lavender essential oil and remix your solution.

Top tip: Your sanitizer will smell like lavender, and will have a thick gel-like appearance due to the Aloe. I recommend you use a squeeze bottle to enjoy your new hand sanitizer.

3.7 Recipe 7

Coconut Oil Recipe

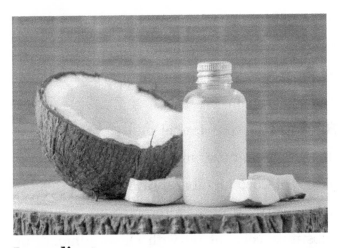

Ingredients:

- 5 ml of liquid coconut oil
- ½ cup of clean tap water
- 20 ml of Alcohol
- 5 drops of cinnamon essential oil
- Bowl
- Measuring cup
- Spoon
- Filter
- Clear Bottle
- Labeling materials

Directions:

Step 1: Pour the fresh water into a bowl, add Alcohol, and mix properly.

Step 2: Add 5ml of coconut oil to your mixture

Step 3: Whisk your solution properly.

Step 4: Add 5 drops of cinnamon essential oil and shake again.

Step 5: Use your funnel and store your new homemade sanitizer in a spray container.

Top tip: Coconut oil is always readily available at grocery stores. Alternatively, you can substitute coconut oil with Olive, Almond, or Peach Oil.

3.8 Recipe 8

Peppermint Homemade Hand Sanitizer

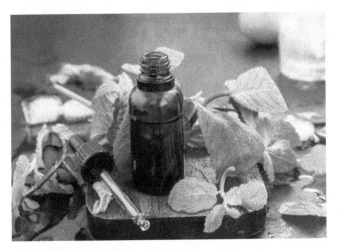

Ingredients:

- 10 drops of peppermint essential oil
- ½ cup of Alcohol or Alcohol tincture
- 5 drops of peach essential oil
- 1 tablespoon of vitamin E
- Bowl
- Measuring cup
- Spoon
- Filter

- Clear Bottle
- Labeling materials

Directions

Step 1: Pour your alcohol tincture into a bowl

Step 2: Add 5 drops of Vitamin E to your solution and mix properly

Step 3: Whisk your solution properly.

Step 4: Add 10 drops of peppermint essential oil and reshake.

Top tip: If you want your homemade hand sanitizer in a spray-able liquid form, ensure the ratio of Alcohol to essential oil is 2:1. However, to get a more gel-like sanitizer, the mixture should be in the ratio of 1:1

3.9 Recipe 9

The Cinnamon Homemade Hand Sanitizer

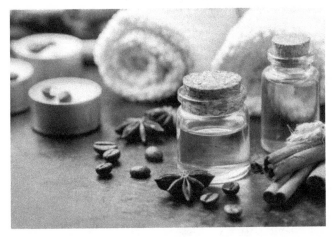

Ingredients

- 10 drops of Cinnamon essential oil;
- 5 drops of tea tree essential oil
- 3 tablespoons of Aloe Vera gel
- **On request:** 1 tablespoon of vitamin E
- Bowl
- Measuring cup
- Spoon
- Filter
- Clear Bottle

- Labeling materials

Directions

Step 1: Pour a 1/3 cup of Aloe gel into 2/3 water, and use your spoon to mix thoroughly.

Step 2: Add 10 drops of cinnamon essential Oil

Step 3: Add a teaspoon of Vitamin E (Helps soften the skin)

Top tip: Essential Oils are not soluble in water, so don't mix well. Ensure you shake the mixture thoroughly or use your whisk.

Step 4: Pour carefully into your clear bottle and label correctly.

3.10 Recipe 10

Hydrogen Peroxide Homemade

Hand Sanitizer

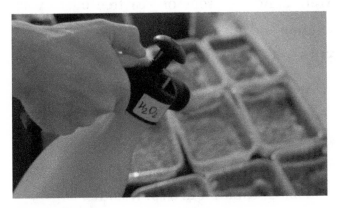

Ingredients

- 150ml of distilled water
- 1 teaspoon of Hydrogen Peroxide
- 5 drops of Tea tree Oil
- 5 drops of Lavender extract
- Bowl
- Measuring cup
- Spoon
- Filter
- Clear Bottle
- Labeling materials

Directions

Step 1: Pour 150ml of distilled water into a bowl, then add 1 tablespoon of Hydrogen peroxide

Step 2: Add 5 drops of Tea tree oil to your solution and mix properly

Step 3: Whisk your solution properly.

Step 4: Add 10 drops of Lavender oil to mask the smell of Hydrogen peroxide, and shake again.

Step 5: Use your funnel to pour your homemade sanitizer in a spray bottle.

Top tip: The Hydrogen peroxide sanitizer has a ton of impressive functions. Besides being an exceptional hand sanitizer, you can also use this solution to disinfect surfaces. I recommend you first try it on a small portion of your furniture.

Now that you've gotten a peek at our coveted recipes, let's have a small recap.

1. Get your ingredients together and ready for use.

2. Mix the suitable ingredients correctly, using appropriate measurements.

3. Pour all ingredients accordingly together in your bowl and mix thoroughly with a spoon. You can use a whisk if you choose to add 1 or 2 essential oils.

4. Sanitize your bottles with leftover Alcohol and leave to air dry.

5. Pour your hand sanitizer into the bottles using a funnel to avoid wastage.

6. Ensure you label your containers correctly to avoid accidental ingestion.

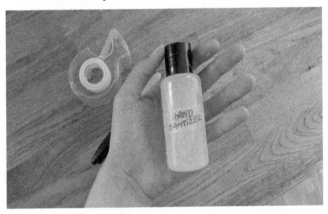

Important note: Alcohols are safe ingredients for hand sanitizers. They naturally don't have any damaging effects on the skin. However, excess use can cause irritation and cracks in the skin.

Chapter 4

4.1 Safety

How safe is your homemade Sanitizer?

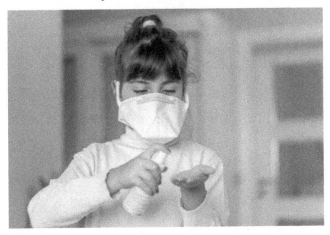

Between the exclusive recipes and the priceless tips we offer, you must have realized making your hand sanitizer at home is incredibly easy. You're not wrong! It is. However, you just have to be extremely cautious, so you don't ruin the recipes. In this section, our primary goal is to guide you through safety precautions when creating your Sanitizer. Staying safe doesn't have to be complicated.

Before you jump into the first step of your favorite recipe, your priority should be ensuring your tools and equipment are properly sterilized. If not, you may end up tainting the potency of your hand sanitizer.

Simply mixing Aloe and Alcohol in a container isn't enough to make a valid hand sanitizer. Some recipes are more complex than others, and their ingredients may not be readily available. You may need to go to the local drug store or grocery shop before you start preparing those unique recipes. Nevertheless, whether your recipe has 5 or 100 ingredients, ensure you mix them using the correct ratios.

You may prefer a complex recipe to a simpler one. Regardless of your choice, some of the ingredients in your preferred recipe could be dangerous, especially when you don't use them in their correct proportion.

So what happens when you use don't use a wrong ingredient, or you don't get the accurate proportions?

- Firstly, your homemade sanitizer may not be as effective as it could be. Ultimately, you'll be at a disadvantage fighting off harmful bacteria, especially since your faulty hand sanitizer can't effectively kill most of the germs you come in contact with.

- Dangerous ingredients in your recipe like alcohol, hydrogen peroxide, and some essential oils can irritate the skin, cause allergic reactions, burns, and severe injury.

- You stand at a higher risk of inhaling hazardous chemicals, which could lead to respiratory problems.

Top tip: I recommend you strictly follow the rules and guidelines when you cook up a recipe for your homemade hand sanitizer, especially if you're in a home with children. Children may be vulnerable to some ingredients, and this could lead to more extreme injuries.

4.2 Where should you keep your Homemade Sanitizer?

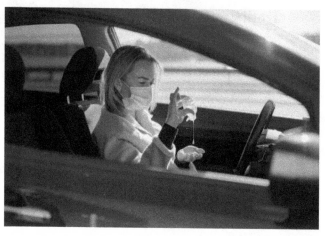

It's no secret that you need a proper place to store items, especially if you have little kids running around the house. But for hand sanitizers, things are a bit different. To reiterate, hand sanitizers are the second-best option after hand washing. So naturally, you should use your hand sanitizer when there's no available sink to wash your hands.

We've come up with ingenious places to store your new homemade Sanitizer. Hand sanitizers are not very active on filthy and greasy hands, so your priority should be storing them in locations where you can't wash your hands immediately.

I recommend you store your hand sanitizer in your car and shelves all around your house, especially in places that kids can't easily access.

Top Tip: According to the World Health Organization (WHO). Before you start using your homemade hand sanitizer, allow your Sanitizer to sit for at least 3 days. This ensures your Sanitizer has enough time to eliminate any contaminant, or germs that may have entered during the preparation process.

Conclusion

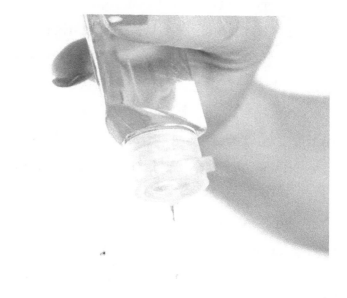

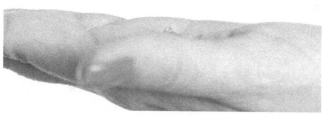

Compared to commercial hand sanitizers, homemade sanitizers represent excellent value for their price. 2019 was a remarkable year for homemade hand sanitizer recipes, especially since there was a significant increase in people appreciating the incredible benefits of a homemade sanitizer. 2020 is going to experience even more success. With new and innovative recipes coming into light every day, the demand for homemade sanitizer recipes is only going to go higher.

With all the new strains of bacteria and viruses that are coming up in the world today, having our homemade sanitizer recipe book is an invaluable advantage.

Like most products, homemade sanitizers have their pros and cons. However, the pros outweigh the cons substantially. They don't occupy much room in your bag, they are super easy to travel with, and they give you a tremendous fighting chance against germs.

FAQ

Question: Can I use vodka as my alcohol ingredient?

Answer: If you have an enormous reserve of vodka, then I have bad news for you. Although vodka is a potent drink, it doesn't have the same effect on germs. According to the CDC, your hand sanitizer needs to have at least 60% alcohol to eliminate bacteria successfully. Unfortunately, Tito, the manufacturer of vodka, confirmed that most vodka is only 40% alcohol (80 proof).

So if you use vodka to make a homemade sanitizer, it won't be very useful.

Question: Is your homemade Sanitizer safe for Kids?

Answer: Children are usually attracted to attractive, sweet-smelling, and flashy objects. With the recipes in your arsenal, your new homemade hand sanitizer is bound to meet one of these requirements. So if you're in a home with children, owning a homemade hand sanitizer can be a considerable risk.

Home sanitizer is not safe for kids. Ingesting hand sanitizers can lead to poisoning, especially if alcohol is your main ingredient. I recommend you store your hand sanitizer in places that aren't easily accessible to children.

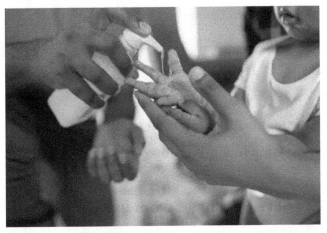

According to a recent study, The United States received over 80,000 cases arising from hand sanitizer poisoning among children during 2011 – 2015 alone.

Question: Can You Drink Homemade Hand Sanitizer?

Answer: The active alcohol ingredient in hand sanitizers may seem inviting to some people, especially teenagers and adults who may intentionally gulp sanitizers to get drunk. On the contrary, drinking your homemade

Sanitizer is not a good idea. Ingesting a handful of your Sanitizer can only cause alcohol poisoning, which can be life-threatening.

Your homemade hand Sanitizer is only safe when it is used as directed.

If you have young children at home, I recommend they use hand sanitizers under the supervision of a grown-up.

So where do you go from here?

As you know, the world is constantly evolving, and likewise, recipes for homemade sanitizers come to light. New recipes emerge, and the techniques and steps change.

There's always something new to learn. So what you learned here is just the beginning.

Always remember to stay up to date on new recipes and fun facts.

Let me know how our recipes work for you.

Thank you so much for sticking it with me this far!

I can't wait to see you again soon!